Health Benefits of PROBIOTICS

A Health Learning Handbook

Dr. S.K. Dash
Dr. Allan N. Spreen
Dr. Beth M. Ley

BL Publications
Temecula, CA

BL Publications, Temecula, CA 92692 1-877-BOOKS11

Dash, S.K. 1942-

Health Benefits of Probiotics/Dr. S.K. Dash, Dr. Allan N. Spreen, Dr. Beth M. Ley.--1st ed.

p. cm. -- "A Health Learning Handbook"

Includes bibliographical references and index.

ISBN: 1-890766-10-0

1. Intestines--Microbiology. 2. Microorganisms-Therapeutic use. 3. Dietary supplements. 4.Gastrointestinal system--Diseases--Alternative treatment. I. Spreen, Allan. II. Ley, Beth M. III. Title. IV. Series.

QR171.I6 D37 1999
616'.014--dc21

Printed in the United States of America

First edition, November 1999

This book is not intended as medical advise. It's purpose is solely educational.

Credits:
Cover Design and Typesetting: BL Publications
Proofreading: Rachel Boyer, Virginia Simpson-Magruder

Table of Contents

Foreword

The book, "Health Benefits of Probiotics" is very informative and is an educational tool for the general public and even for college students pursuing interest in food science, nutrition, bacteriology and related areas.

The book covers current research on health benefits of probiotics on digestive disorders, cholesterol, immune system, yeast infection, ulcer, cancer, acne, and much more.

As the use of probiotics grows, the public needs more and more information on probiotics, and this book effectively provides this.

Dr. S.K. Dash has been a pioneer in the field of probiotics for the past 25 years. He and his associates have tried to put this book in a brief, easy to read format for the general public.

I commend Dr. Dash for this venture.

Prof. S.C. Panda, M.D. FAIID, FAMS

Ex-visiting Professor, The Rockefeller University, NY
Retired Professor and HOD Biochemistry and DMET and Additional Secretary Health and F.W., Dept., Govt. of Orissa

Introduction

Probiotics may be a new word to some of you. It may sound familiar, however, as most people know what antibiotics are - drugs used to kill bacteria in the body. Probiotics are the opposite, as their purpose is to promote friendly bacteria in the body.

The word *probiotics* actually means *for life.* It includes not only the commonly known lactic acid bacteria (found in yogurt), but all naturally occurring beneficial bacteria in our intestinal tract.

The amount of bacteria present in the digestive system is so huge, they are counted in powers of 10; 10^3 is 1,000 and 10^6 is 1,000,000. In the esophagus, the numbers are 10^3 to 10^6 per gram of contents. In the small intestine there are about 10^3 to 10^6 bacteria per gram, and this increases in the large intestine or colon to 10^8 to 10^{11}. In the feces, 10 or 20% of the weight consists of bacteria, most of which are anaerobic; that is, they can grow without oxygen.

Acidophilus, while a prominent player in the effort to maintain human intestinal health, is actually only one of over 400 species different of bacteria in our intestinal tracts. (Bagchi) In fact, there are over 200 strains just of acidophilus. (Accessory Nutrients, p. 360)

These organisms are also called intestinal flora, gut flora, or microflora. To distinguish the good ones from the others, the term "probiotics" arose to prominence in the nutritional science world.

Throughout history cultures (of people) have benefited from the use of cultures (of probiotics). Whether the growth of these bacteria came from sour cream, cheese, kefir, yogurt, sauerkraut or kim chee (fermented cabbage), miso (fermented soy), or whatever, there has been prominent use of probiotics, even by those who didn't know why it helped - only that it did.

Even prior to our first breath we were exposed to probiotics. On the way through the birth canal a normal-delivery child gets dosed with the bacteria of the mother's vaginal tract. The prominent normal organisms in this area, in a healthy woman, called Doderlein's bacilli, are recognized to be L. acidophilus. This starts colonization right from the very beginning into the infant's GI tract, and may be one of several reasons that caesarean-section babies have a bit of a tougher time than normal births. There are also differences (which you might expect) in the make-up of the intestinal flora between breast-fed and formula-fed babies. (Haenel, Rotimi, Stark)

Probiotic History and Development

Almost a century ago, Russian researcher Dr. E. Metchnikoff became convinced that yogurt contained the organisms necessary to protect the intestine from the damaging effects of other bacteria that putrefied there. His belief was that toxins produced by ""bad guy"" bugs in this process could be handled by the presence of "good guy" lactic acid bacteria in the yogurt. (Metchnikoff)

His work was basically ignored by the conventional mainstream. Apparently, it was believed that a solid step toward good health could not be that simple (or should not be that cheap!), so funds for generating a body of confirming evidence were not forth coming. That lack of evidence is rapidly changing.

In the 1950's the first probiotic product was approved as a drug and sold by a major pharmaceutical company. However, it quickly disappeared from the market as antibiotics gained popularity as the miracle drug of the time. But the growing use and abuse of antibiotics is rendering them helpless to fight bacterial infections, and increasing the importance of probiotics as a solution.

Effects of Probiotics

There are (at least) seven ways live bacteria products benefit the body:

1. Normalize the intestinal tract.

2. Suppress growth of pathogenic and putrefactive bacteria.

3. Increase resistance against infections.

4. Produce lactic acid, acetic acid, butyric acid and natural antibiotics.

5. Manufacture B complex and other vitamins: (Hughes, Noda, McDonough)

Biotin	Thiamine (B-l)
Riboflavin (B-2)	Pyridoxine (B-6)
Pantothenic acid (B-5)	Vitamin K

6. Form a favorable medium for growth of bifidus bacteria.

7. Produce hydrogen peroxide.

8. Miscellaneous applications:

- Support and strengthen overall immunity
- Produce their own antibacterial substances against invading organisms
- Increase the over-all digestive abilities of the GI tract
- Provide resistance against damage from pollutants and radiation

Enhance Nutrient Absorption

Many nutrients are dependent upon probiotic cultures for adequate digestion and proper utilization. Though we may get nutrients from a variety of sources, absorption of optimum amounts may depend in large part on the overall health of the intestines and their resident 'guests'.

Absorption of the minerals calcium, zinc, iron, manganese, copper and phosphorus is enhanced with the use of probiotics. (McDonough)

Foods fermented with probiotics have proteins that are more easily absorbed. Amino acids, the protein building blocks, are also more available in fermented foods like yogurt, when compared to milk. (Alm)

The huge numbers of bacteria in the colon actively affect the other constituents of the gut. These are mostly harmless bacteria which tend to reduce the number of pathogenic organisms entering the gut. Without these beneficial bacteria, we are much more susceptible to intestinal infection, cancer and other things to be discussed later.

The use of antibiotics and other drugs inhibits the amount of vitamins supplied by the bacteria, increasing our need for these nutrients. Bacteria also digest small constituents of dietary fiber, enabling them to be absorbed. Another function of intestinal bacteria is to break down bile pigments and bile acids.

Without a steady supply of probiotics in the gut, we cannot properly benefit from these intestinal flora.

Probiotics Are Extremely Safe

It is rare in today's high-tech, magic-bullet world, to find any therapeutic agent that truly does no harm. Almost all prescription drugs have a long list of side effects and toxicities. Common over-the-counter aspirin is well known to cause stomach and intestinal irritation, severe bleeding, and other problems. Even very high doses of certain nutrient supplements can be toxic.

Even plain water can be toxic, if you take too much of it. However, probiotics, as a class of nutrient supplement, has to rank right down there at the bottom with water. In fact, it is much easier to take too little. Daily dosage range suggestions are listed between one and ten billion cells. Less than that actually may not be enough to have the culture set up housekeeping and hang around. Aggressive efforts to overdo it may only produce mild GI disturbances, and true safety issues seem to be non-existent.

Oral administration of probiotics are well tolerated and proven to be safe in 143 human clinical trials and no adverse effects were reported in any of the total 7,526 individuals studied during 1961-1998. (Naidu)

Individuals sensitive to milk products seem to tolerate dairy sources of probiotics, though there are alternatives to dairy sources. Lactose intolerant individuals can significantly increase their tolerance to dairy products with the use of probiotic supplements. (Saltzman, Kolars; Kim and Gilliland; Savaiano)

You are what you eat is no joke. The fuel for the machine is the main determinant of how it will run. If your GI tract is toxic, maldigestive or malabsorptive, the nutrients in your diet are handled poorly. This can allow borderline deficiencies to cause overt symptoms of illness. How your body handles the food it is fed, good or bad, can have a major impact on how you feel.

Probiotic cultures are a major component of the interior of our digestive systems - intimately involved in nearly every process. Be it detoxifying, digestion, absorption, or even producing nutrients by themselves, we will see that probiotic cultures are truly the all-around "good-guys" of our insides.

From the day we are born until the day we die we need large quantities of probiotics within us. Sadly, in this world of refined foods and quick-fix medications, it is much easier to kill these guys than to keep them in residence.

However, if you educate yourself and take advantage of the sources available to us, you and your family can reap the rewards of this important nutritional supplement without a lot of effort.

Probiotics and Digestive Disorders

The digestive system is an involved system starting in the mouth and ending at the anus. As food and beverages travel this route, food is broken down for easier digestion by salivary glands, the gall bladder, liver and the pancreas.

Intestinal flora, such as acidophilus, are an important aspect of a healthy digestive tract. The warm body temperature, moisture and ample food provide an ideal medium for bacteria to thrive. The further down the GI tract, the more bacteria are present. The upper intestine should have fewer bacteria than 10,000 per ml. The bulk of the weight of the feces is bacteria.

The bacteria count is reduced in the upper part of the GI tract by strong stomach acids. Those who lack sufficient amounts of acid are more apt to suffer bacterial overgrowth, with yeast cells among them. The growth of bacteria is highest in the colon and rectum, and lowest in the duodenum.

Harmful bacteria not only interfere with the absorption of nutrients, they produce toxins that injure intestinal walls, interfering with the absorption of nutrients and water.

A high-fiber diet stimulates peristalsis, moving the food through within a day or so. The longer that fecal matter remains in the digestive system, the greater the chances for harmful carcinogens to build up. When digestion is normal, with the assistance of healthy probiotic levels, harmful bacteria are less likely to cause damage to the digestive tract.

In addition to constipation, a malfunctioning digestive tract can produce a variety of painful and unpleasant disorders, most of which are related to diet and lifestyle. These include appendicitis, Crohn's disease, diverticulitis, gallbladder disease, gastritis, gastroenteritis, hemorrhoids, hiatal hernia, irritable bowel syndrome, pancreatitis, ulcerative colitis and other conditions.

No one has perfect digestion, or at least, it is extremely rare. We all experience heartburn, burping, bloating, and gas from time to time (even if we blame it on the dog). A positive over-all effect of probiotics is that the organisms scavenge indigestible molecules throughout the GI tract. They also suppress putrefaction of foods, and displace other bacteria that tend to putrefy. (Hida, O'Sullivan, Gorbach)

Probiotics produce enzymes which help breakdown and digest the food we eat. This reduces bloating, improves utilization of nutrients, reduces gas and putrefaction, and much more.

Almost everyone can benefit from probiotic supplementation, especially if any chronic illness is involved. Few people have been around very long without running into refined diets, which have a stressful effect on our GI tracts.

Heart Burn

Even minor 'heart burn' symptoms commonly clear quickly with administration of probiotics. Antacids should be avoided as they are detrimental because we need acid in our digestive systems. Its presence is not the result of some mistake on the part of Mother Nature. It is vitally important, and we want to keep it there, not neutralize it. If symptoms can be alleviated using something far safer, and still allow our normal acid to remain, what could be better?

Food Allergies

Food allergies (sensitivities) can interfere with proper digestion (as anyone with a serious sensitivity can tell you). Probiotic research data support its use in the management of this difficult disorder. (Majamaa)

The gastrointestinal microflora is an important constituent of the gut mucosal defense barrier. Lactobacillus promotes local antigen-specific immune responses (particularly in the IgA class), prevents permeability defects, and confers controlled antigen absorption. Probiotic bacteria may promote endogenous barrier mechanisms in patients with atopic dermatitis and food allergy, and by alleviating intestinal inflammation, may act as a useful tool in the treatment of food allergy. (Majamaa)

Lactose (Milk Sugar) Intolerance

Lactose intolerance is believed to be experienced by an estimated 30 million Americans. The digestive enzyme, lactase, needed to digest lactose is not present. Symptoms include bloating, gas, stomach cramps, diarrhea and other intestinal discomforts after consuming dairy products.

Products containing lactase are helpful as are probiotics. (Kim, Hove) The bacteria don't even have to be consumed every time the dairy product is eaten, and digestion is still improved. The degree of improvement is somewhat dose-dependent.

Turkish researchers who conducted a double-blind, cross over study, reported that probiotics appear to regulate the nonspecific immune response differently in healthy and hypersensitive subjects. This is seen as an immunostimulatory effect in healthy subjects, and as a down-regulation of inflammatory response in milk-hypersensitive subjects. (Pelto)

Intestinal disorders (inflammatory bowel disease), medications (antibiotics and antiinflammatories), and surgery can also reduce lactase production in the body. Even though it may only be temporary, these individuals can also greatly benefit from probiotic supplementation.

Diarrheal Diseases

Probiotics are intimately involved with intestinal health. Diarrhea is an indication that the state of intestinal health has been compromised, whether due to toxins, pathological bacteria, rancidity, medication reaction, or something else. Whatever the cause, it is a common finding that the probiotic population is reduced.

Whether the diarrhea or the altered flora is the proverbial chicken or the egg is subject to conjecture. Either way the use of a good probiotic supplement can significantly improve the outcome of diarrheal disease. Whether the problem has to do with the use of antibiotics, which kill both good and bad bacteria, or the mere presence of too many bad bacteria, like in salmonella or shigella-induced diarrhea, probiotics can help. (Gotz, Hitchins, Alm, Clements)

Many forms of probiotics themselves have antimicrobial activity of multiple mechanisms. (Modler) Researchers at the University of Nebraska established at least three separate chemicals produced by acidophilus (using DDS® from UAS Laboratories) that can kill other bacteria:

Acidophilin (a natural antibiotic effective against Strep, Staph and E. coli bugs),

Lactic acid, and

Hydrogen peroxide. (Sehnert)

Also, toxic by-products like ammonia can be decreased by the presence of probiotics, which inhibit organisms that produce this chemical. (Modler)

This becomes significant not only in helping with the control of diarrhea, but also in the treatment of ulcers.

For world travelers some reassuring information concerning the constant menace of traveler's diarrhea has emerged. Studies as far as Mexico, Guatemala, and Nepal showed remarkable improvement over expected outbreaks after using probiotics. In fact, with just two capsules a day (DDS ® from UAS Laboratories) an expected incidence of 25-30% was less than 3% in a population of

70 participants. (Sehnert)

Prolonged diarrhea responds just as well with high doses of probiotics as with drugs designed to slow down the GI tract. The former solution is far safer, since artificially inhibiting the movement of the intestinal tract (peristalsis) allows more time for absorption of toxins in the large intestine.

Traveler's Trots: Three studies conducted in 1987-1989, consisting of a total of 70 individuals travelling to Guatamala, Mexico and Nepal demonstrated substantial protection against digestive disorders among those who took two capsules DDS® Acidophilus before breakfast each day starting one week before departure and throughout the trip. The incidence of diarrhea was only two individuals, whereas the usual incidence is 35-30%. (Sehnert)

Constipation

It may be hard to believe that something good for diarrhea could also be good for constipation. Such can be the case, however, when you are using something that 'normalizes' the GI tract, instead of just forcing a response to a particular symptom.

Probiotics have a history, from a number of sources, of having an beneficial effect on problems with constipation. (Bagchi; Alm,1984; Salminen) Finnish researchers clearly demonstrated its ability to lower colonic pH balancing intestinal microecology and normalize intestinal transit and therefore, effectively relieve constipation in humans. (Salminen)

Reestablishing and maintaining the beneficial bacterial environment in the gastrointestinal tract can pay dividends or result in symptoms that don't seem related.

Bad Breath

Even bad breath (halitosis) can involve abnormal

intestinal flora as a significant part of its cause. Colonization of upper portions of the GI tract by putrefying organisms can have effects on a person's breath odor. Years of bothersome symptoms have been successfully handled once the status of the microenvironment has been addressed. (Sehnert, Atkinson-Barr)

In addition to bad breath, canker sores, belching, bloating, and flatulence can also result from abnormal intestinal flora.

Gastritis and Ulcers

Spicy food and stress are no longer receiving all the blame for causing stomach and intestinal ulcers. Evidence now points towards a new cause: The bacterium Helicobacter pylori (H. pylori). More than half of the population is infected with it. The elderly and people in developing countries are at most risk for infection. H. pylori has also been implicated in other illnesses as well. These include: Gastritis, skin disorders, autoimmune disorders, fatigue, growth retardation and heart disease. (Fieforek, Blaser)

Unfortunately, this little guy is tough to kill. The bug survives stomach acid without difficulty. Single antibiotics aren't enough. A triple regimen of antibiotic drugs is required for its extermination. To make things worse, H pylori infection is often accompanied by an overgrowth of the yeast, Candida Albicans, which actually serves to protect H. pylori from heat, acid, dehydration, and even antibiotics. (Siavoshi)

Though not present in all earlier cases, the association is made by the fact that the reoccurance of ulcers is much slower with probiotic treatment. The hardy H. pylori organism, requiring three or four drugs to adequately kill it, causes havoc upon the rest of the body. Few other bacteria are this advanced in protecting themselves so they are more easily destroyed. This also allows more yeast to set up, which in turn protect the H. pylori better.

The standard protocol is now a triple regimen of antibiotics and probiotics. (NIH, Lykova, Alba)

Probiotics are beneficial in at least two ways:

1. Probiotics protect against the downside of antibiotics. While you're killing the harmful bacteria, you want to keep reestablishing the friendly bacteria. This can be done both during and after the drug therapy. Especially after the cessation of the antibiotics an additional week or two of a beneficial culture of organisms is recommended. (Lykova, Alba)

2. Probiotics specifically have an affect against H. pylori. Selected strains of L. acidophilus were found to inhibit the growth of H. pylori in the laboratory. (Midolo)

It was shown that the probiotic strains that produced lactic acid, helped slow down the H. pylori. What was even better news was the fact that some other mechanism, as yet undetermined, was also at work to fight the ulcer bug, since the most inhibition was caused by strains that did not produce the most acid. (Midolo)

This ulcer bug (H. pyrolie) is known to cause irritation of the stomach lining (gastritis), which may or may not progress to ulceration. The goal in prevention of problems would be to acquire as much protection as possible for the stomach lining. Not only would you want that protection to be something non-toxic, but also something that can withstand the environment of the intestinal tract, while actively doing something as a protective agent.

Probiotic cultures are able to do just that. By suppressing putrefaction mechanisms, scavenging indigestible molecules, and helping to control the proper acidity level, probiotics are an important line of defense against all sorts of invasions. (Mitsuoka, Modler)

Inflammatory Bowel Diseases

The most common forms of Inflammatory bowel disease (IBD) are ulcerative colitis and Crohn's disease.

Ulcerative Colitis

Ulcerative colitis is a chronic, episodic, inflammatory condition of the large intestine and rectum. It is characterized by watery diarrhea containing blood, mucus and pus, severe abdominal pain, fever, chills, anemia and weight loss. Ulcerative colitis is associated with an increased risk for colon cancer.

Antiinflammatory steriods are commonly used to to control symptoms, but with only marginal success. Researchers in Germany have demonstrated the benefits of probiotic therapy for ulcerative colitis. In light of the hypothesis that the intestinal environment may contribute to the pathophysiology of ulcerative colitis, a double-blind trial was conducted to test the effects of probiotic supplementation with an oral preparation of non-pathogenic E. coli.

One hundred twenty patients with inactive ulcerative colitis were either given a oral probiotic treatment or an oral preparation of viable E. coli for 12 weeks to examine their efficacy in preventing a relapse of the disease.

Relapse rates were 11.3% under probiotic treatment and 16.0% under E. coli. Even though the relapse times were similar, tolerability to the probiotic treatment was excellent and no serious adverse effects were reported. The researchers concluded that probiotic supplementation appears to offer another option for maintenance therapy of ulcerative colitis. (Kruis)

Canadian researchers recently reported on their findings on inflammatory bowel disease and colitis. They found that L. acidophilus repopulated the colonic luman which reduced pathogenic bacteria in the colon and therefore, prevented colitis. (Madsen)

Crohn's Disease

Crohn's disease is a chronic inflammatory bowel disease usually affecting the ileum or colon. It is characterized by frequent attacks of diarrhea, severe abdominal pain, nausea, fever, chills, weakness, loss of appetite and weight loss. The disease is often confused as ulcerative colitis as the symptoms are so similar.

Antibiotics and antiinflammatory steriods are commonly used to to control symptoms. Surgical removal of the diseased portion of the bowel provides relief but reoccurance after surgery is likely.

Bifidobacteria levels decrease in Crohn's Disease

Researchers in France have reported that digestive bacterial microflora and an exaggerated reaction of the intestinal immune system play a major role in the pathogenesis of Crohn's disease.

Bacterial enzyme activities, especially beta-D-galactosidase, are decreased in Crohn's disease patients. Bifidobacteria numbers were significantly reduced in patients of active Crohn's disease. Beta-D-Galactosidase activity and Bifidobacteria counts were significantly correlated. The reduction in Bifidobacteria is responsible for decreased beta-D-galactosidase activity. The researchers stated that as Bifidobacteria are regarded as beneficial, oral administration of probiotics and prebiotics that promote their growth might have potential therapeutic interest. (Favier)

Other researchers have also reported that therapeutic options for Crohn's disease include specific immunomodulatory therapy with cytokines or cytokine antibodies. Maintenance therapy may be performed with probiotics and antioxidants. (von Ritter)

All antibiotics adversely affect acidophilus, bifidus, and other beneficial bacteria. Such treatments usually promote the growth of yeast, thus causing additional complications.

The benefits of probiotics extend far beyond just fighting yeast in the treatment of IBD. Certain strains of L. acidophilus have been shown not to adversely affect the mucus protection mechanism of intestinal walls, and are therefore safe in helping to prevent ulcerative colitis. (Bagchi)

An article in the *Journal of the American Medical Association* in 1996 concluded that probiotics (called bio-therapeutic agents) use a multitude of mechanisms in treating intestinal diseases and should be explored in greater detail for such purposes. Advantages listed included low risk, presumed low cost, and likely existence of multiple mechanisms of action for a single agent-not to mention the fact that probiotics "may offer an alternative to conventional antimicrobials to which many pathogenic microorganisms eventually develop resistance." (Elmer)

Taking inadequate amounts of probiotics decreases their survival chances. Remember, they are needed by the billions. 'Overdosing' is merely a matter of' expense, not a health danger.

Despite continued uncertainty about the cause of inflammatory bowel diseases, recent advances nourish the hope for further improvement of the control of disease activity and a better quality of life.

Probiotics and Antibiotic Therapy

Antibiotics are a class of drugs capable of inhibiting bacterial growth or of killing them outright. They are only available by prescription - and for good reason. The casual use of antibiotics often leads to the development of adaptation or resistance in the invading organism. This can happen when insufficient doses are used or when a sufficient dose is not used until the conclusion of the infection.

Antibiotics also have side effects - some of them are very serious. Many people are allergic (some with even life-threatening reactions) to penicillin and other members of the penicillin family.

Antibiotics can cause side effects because they upset the normal balance of microorganisms in the intestines and vagina. Antibiotics get rid of all bacteria in the body - not just the undesirables. This allows pathogens to take advantage of the breach in the body's defenses, particularly yeast.

Candida albicans is a normal inhabitant of the body, but without adequate levels of friendly bacteria to keep it in check, it rapidly spreads, frequently causing infections of the vagina, bowel, and throat, producing antigens and toxins that can cause neurological or endocrinological problems. (See more on this in the next section)

This bacterial disruption can also reduce the availability of several of the B vitamins, and also Vitamin A, folic acid, zinc and magnesium.

If you must go on antibiotics - meaning there is no other alternative to restore your health, a high dose regimen of probiotics should be used immediately following to replenish all that were lost. They should not be used at the same time as the antibiotics are likely to greatly diminish the benefits of the probiotics.

Probiotics and Yeast Infection/Candidiasis

Bacteria, of course, are not the only microscopic organism naturally occurring in the body. There are all sorts of one-celled microbes in nature, and they can be friends, enemies, or neutral players. Yeast is a single-celled fungus that is usually rounded in appearance, but can change its shape under certain circumstances, sometimes forming budding projections.

The existence of Candida albicans, is normally kept in check by adequate levels of probiotics which compete with yeast in many areas, including habitat and many food sources. This competition permits us to live a 'truce-like' existence with them.

Many things can disrupt the probiotics that do not adversely affect yeast, and this allows the latter to increase their numbers substantially while their adversaries are weakened, for whatever reason. Antibiotics, synthetic hormones, other drugs, non-breathing clothing or cosmetics that plug skin pores, diseases, and other things can give these opportunists a chance to get out of hand. The result of this is symptoms ranging from local infections to a complete take over of the entire body, which for obvious reasons is much more difficult to get rid of.

Local Yeast Infections

Vaginal yeast infections are unfortunately well known to a majority of women. Itching, irritation and cheesy discharge are the annoying symptoms indicating the return of Candida albicans to the vaginal area.

Young children (and more and more older ones) often get yeast overgrowth, appearing as white patches on their tongues. This is called thrush.

Men are not immune, either, as yeast may be responsible for red inflammation and itching in the inner thigh areas, but the female anatomy makes them the worst victims. Yeast may cause its misery not only in the vaginal area, but also in the breasts of lactating women, where it can be considerably painful. It also seems that once an infection has set in, reoccurance of an overgrowth is easy and often - even after successful treatment. The only way to prevent this is by maintaining optimal levels of probiotic bacteria at all times.

Avoiding sugar and refined carbohydrates (which feed the yeast) is also important as is avoiding antibiotics. It seems that the gentle good guys tend to die more quickly than the ones we want to get rid of. They aren't as well-trained as the diseased bacteria in the microscopic guerrilla-warfare of withstanding the onslaught of ever-stronger antibiotics. In fact, the mere presence of invading organisms like triehomonas (T. vaginalis) may by itself lower the concentration of benevolent bacteria. (McGrory)

The standard medical treatment for these infections consists of a 'cidal' agent that preferentially kills yeast which certainly makes some degree of sense. You have too many bad guys; you have an agent that kills 'em. .. so what's wrong with this picture?

Sometimes the body's wonderful defenses, once the main invading army is knocked down, can keep the patient symptom-free, and sometimes that army can eventually rebuild. For years in Europe, prior to these fungicidal drugs, women knew to handle yeast infections with vaginal applications of plain yogurt which is loaded with competitive, probiotic bacteria.

Probiotic culture can also be directly applied to the vaginal area, such as by sprinkling it on a moistened tampon, and then inserting it overnight. (Elmer, Hilton)

For oral yeast (thrush), several times a day, open a probiotic capsule and the pour the contents into the mouth. Hold it as long as possible before swallowing. Do not rinse your mouth or drink anything for at least 20 minutes.

Systemic Yeast

Systemic yeast, which is essentially yeast invading the entire body, sometimes called chronic candidiasis, candida-related-complex (CRC), or just candidias for short, is very common. While this is controversial, as most skeptical medical professionals believe that it only rarely occurs among individuals with life-threatening instances of serious immunity problems, such as in AIDS or chemotherapy cases.

The list of symptoms of systemic yeast are very extensive. So extensive, that the patient becomes unbelievable and the problem is then believed to be, by far too many medical professionals, "all in their head." Not only is the disease real, it is debilitating enough that it needs to be taken seriously.

Candidiasis is believed to contribute to food allergies, menstrual problems, depression, impairment of memory and ability to concentrate, and severe fatigue. It may even worsen preexisting autoimmune conditions. It is, however, treatable, and probiotics play a major role in the therapy. (Fitzsimmons)

Systemic yeast treatment involves killing the bad guys (usually orally), reestablishing the good guys (probiotics), and using a few additional therapeutics such as FOS (which is discussed later) to encourage the probiotics to set up housekeeping inside.

William Crook, M.D., a pioneer on this topic, and author of *The Yeast Connection,* has graciously permitted the reprinting of his 'Candida Questionnaire.' If your score is high, you need to finish this book, and then go get his.

To determine whether candidiasis is a potential problem, take the following quiz designed by Dr. Crook.

Candida Questionnaire And Score Sheet

This questionnaire is designed for adults and the scoring system isn't appropriate for children. It lists factors in your medical history which promote the growth of Candida albicans (Section A), and symptoms commonly found in individuals with yeast-connected illness (Section B and C).

For each "Yes" answer in Section A, circle the Point Score in that section. Total your score and record it in the box at the end of the section. Then move on to Sections B and C and score as directed.

Filling out and scoring this questionnaire should help you and your physician evaluate the possible role of candida in contributing to your health problems. Yet it will not provide an automatic "Yes" or "No" answer.

SECTION A: HISTORY

	Point Score
1. Have you taken tetracyclines (Sumycin®, Panmycin®, Vibramycin®, Minocin®, etc.) or other antibiotics for acne or 1 month (or longer)?	35
2. Have you, at any time in your life, taken other "broad spectrum" antibiotics for respiratory, urinary or other infections (for 2 months or longer, or in shorter courses 4 or more times in a 1-year period?)	35
3. Have you taken a broad spectrum antibiotic drug, — including Keflex,® ampicillin, amoxicillin, Ceclor,® Bactrim® and Septra®. Even a single course?	6
4. Have you, at any time in your life, been bothered by persistent prostatitis, vaginitis or other problems affecting your reproductive organs?	25
5. Have you been pregnant... 2 or more times?	5
1 time?	3
6. Have you taken birth control pills...	
For more than 2 years?	15
For 6 months to 2 years?	8
7. Have you taken prednisone, Decadron® or other cortisone-type drugs... For more than 2 weeks	15
For 2 weeks or less?	6
8. Does exposure to perfumes, insecticides, fabric shop odors and other chemicals provoke...	
Moderate to severe symptoms?	20
Mild symptoms?	5
9. Are your symptoms worse on damp, muggy days or in moldy places?	20

10. Have you had athlete's foot, ring worm, "jock itch" or other chronic fungous infections of the skin or nails? Have such infec-

tions been.. .Severe or persistent?	20
Mild to moderate?	10
11. Do you crave sugar?	10
12. Do you crave breads?	10
13. Do you crave alcoholic beverages?	10
14. Does tobacco smoke really bother you?	10

Total Score, Section A ____________

SECTION B: MAJOR SYMPTOMS

For each of your symptoms, enter the appropriate figure in the Point Score column:
If a symptom is occasional or mild, score **3 points**
If a symptom is frequent and/or moderately severe, score **6 points**
If a symptom is severe and/or disabling, score **9 points.**
Add total score and record it in the box at the end of this section.

	Point Score
1. Fatigue or lethargy	______
2. Feeling of being "drained"	______
3. Depression	______
4. Poor memory	______
5. Feeling spacy or "unreal"	______
6. Inability to make decisions	______
7. Numbness, burning or tingling	______
8. Headache	______
9. Muscle aches	______
10. Muscle weakness or paralysis	______
11. Pain and/or swelling in joints	______
12. Abdominal pain	______
13. Constipation and/or diarrhea	______
14. Bloating, belching or intestinal gas	______
15. Troublesome vaginal burning, itching or discharge	______
16. Prostatitis	______
17. Impotence	______
18. Loss of sexual desire or feeling	______
19. Endometriosis or infertility	______
20. Cramps and/or other menstrual irregularities	______
21. Premenstrual tension	______
22. Attacks of anxiety or crying	______
23. Cold hands or feet and/or chilliness	______
24. Shaking or irritable when hungry	______

Total Score, Section B ____________

SECTION C: OTHER SYMPTOMS

For each of your symptoms, enter the appropriate figure in the Point Score column:
If a symptom is occasional or mild, score **1 point**
If a symptom is frequent and/or moderately severe, score **2 points**
If a symptom is severe and/or disabling, score **3 points**
Add total score and record it in the box at the end of this section.

Note: While the symptoms in this section commonly occur in people with yeast-connected illness they are also found in other individuals.

	Point Score
1. Drowsiness	________
2. Irritability or jitteriness	________
3. Incoordination	________
4. Inability to concentrate	________
5. Frequent mood swings	________
6. Insomnia	________
7. Dizziness/loss of balance	________
8. Pressure above ears /feeling of head swelling	________
9. Tendency to bruise easily	________
10. Chronic rashes or itching	________
11. Numbness, tingling	________
12. Indigestion or heartburn	________
13. Food sensitivity or intolerance	________
14. Mucus in stools	________
15. Rectal itching	________
16. Dry mouth or throat	________
17. Rash or blisters in mouth	________
18. Bad breath	________
19. Foot, hair or body odor not relieved by washing	________
20. Nasal congestion or post nasal drip	________
21. Nasal itching	________
22. Sore throat	________
23. Laryngitis, loss of voice	________
24. Cough or recurrent bronchitis	________
25. Pain or tightness in chest	________
26. Wheezing or shortness of breath	________
27. Urinary frequency or urgency	________
28. Burning on urination	________
29. Spots in front of eyes or erratic vision	________
30. Burning or tearing of eyes	________
31. Recurrent infections or fluid in ears	________

32. Ear pain or deafness __________

Total Score, Section C ____________________

Total Score, Section A __________

Total Score, Section B __________

GRAND TOTAL SCORE __________

The Grand Total Score will help you and your physician decide if your health problems are yeast-connected. Scores in women will run higher as 7 items in the questionnaire apply exclusively to women, while only 2 apply exclusively to men.

Yeast-connected health problems are almost certainly present in women with scores **over 180**, and in men with scores **over 140**.

Yeast-connected health problems are probably present in women with scores **over 120**, and in men with scores **over 90.**

Yeast-connected health problems are possibly present in women with scores **over 60**, and in men with scores **over 40.**

With scores of **less than 60** in women and **less than 40** in men, yeasts are less apt to cause health problems.

The following laboratories offer blood tests that can confirm and monitor exposure to candida:

Great Smokies Diagnostic Laboratories
63 Zillicoa Street, Asherville, NC, 28801
800-522-4762

Immunodiagnostic Laboratories
488 McCormick, San Leandro, CA 94577
800-888-1113

Immuno Laboratories
1620 W. Oakland Park Blvd. Ft. Lauderdale, FL 33311
800-231-9197/ 954-486-4500
web site: http:/www.imunolabs.com

CRC Treatment Options

Treatment regimens to adequately control the organism must include dietary changes so that the refined carbohydrates that yeast like best are not supplied. Besides the ingestion of probiotics, a multitude of other agents are considered for making the intestinal environment as receptive as possible so the microflora flourish. Such agents include garlic, various herbs, and fructooligosacharides (FOS), which will be discussed later.

Often a victim of candidiasis has had a long history of antibiotics, synthetic hormones, sugar, junk food, and other negative influences on their bodies. One doesn't get this way in a day or a week and active efforts to kill yeast beyond establishing a population of probiotic organisms are usually in order.

Such treatments can be a program of natural agents, including caprylic acid, grapefruit seed extract, olive leaf extract and/or others, and even prescription medication, such as nystatin fluconazole (Diflucan®), ketoconazole (Nizoral®), itraconazole (Snoranox®), terbinafine (Lamisil®), and possibly others.

An understanding and open-minded physician is needed to treat this disorder. Self-education is very important and can be done by reading *The Yeast Connection*, or other excellent works.

The following is the protocol used by Keith Sehnert, M.D., author of *The Gardin Within* for CRC:

1. Yeast-killing medication: Nystatin powder, U.S.P. is preferred because of its flexible dosage form. It can be taken by mouth; used as a douche; applied as soaks to skin, finger, or toe nails; or mixed with a simple salt solution for application as nose or ear drops.

The average person takes this for 16 weeks. When the antibody levels drop to a normal range as indicated by laboratory testing, the nystatin is stopped. Ketoconazole

(Nizoral, the Janssen Company) is recommended if a patient doesn't respond to nystatin or when that individual has chronic sinusitis or genito-urinary problems such as prostatitus or chronic cystitis.

2. Low sugar, yeast-free diet: Because candida thrives on sugar and simple carbohydrates, a careful diet must be followed. During the first two weeks, patients must also avoid fruits, as they are high in sugar.

A yeast-free diet is required for one week. This means avoiding breads, cakes, cookies and donuts; many cheeses; wine, beer, alcoholic beverages; vinegar and some dried fruits. This is important as even though these yeasts may be only "cousins" of candida there is cross-over sensitivity that can cause reactions. After one week, the individual may try a "challenge dose" by eating some bread, cheese or other foods with yeast. If there is no reaction or problem, these foods may then be resumed. The *Yeast Connection Cookbook* by Dr. Crook is a useful resource.

3. Lactobacillus acidophilus: DDS Acidophilus, marketed by UAS Laboratories is recommended because of its potency, quality and effectiveness. It is also less expensive than many competitive products.

4. Mineral, vitamin and other nutritional supplements: Because patients are on a restricted diet, supplemental vitamin/mineral tablets or capsules are recommended as is additional Vitamin C, calcium and magnesium. Note: Excess zinc is believed to promote the growth of candida and should be avoided. Caprylic acid (a fatty acid derived from coconut oil) is also recommended because of its anti-fungal qualities. There are many acceptable brands.

5. Other recommendations: Avoid antibiotics (unless absolutely necessary), oral contraceptive tablets and corticosteriods while on treatment (and use them with caution after recovery!). Because of the high incidence of allergies, immune globulin testing for common foods is a good idea. If an individual suspects common foods known to cause allergies such as dairy products or wheat, they should be eliminated from the diet.

One should also increase exercise, practice stress management, modify negative lifestyles and improve the work and home environment. When necessary, psychological and spiritual counseling is provided.

6. Other therapies: Although I do not use all of them on a routine basis, other therapeutic agents include herbal teas such as taheebo and mathake, garlic, and essential fatty acids.

The factors that set the stage for this yeast infection the first time can occur again. There is no "quick fix" for CRC. The responsibility for healthy living lies with each individual and they must continue to be on guard as an Activated Patient

Probiotics and Cholesterol

Even those familiar with the use of probiotics for all sorts of gastrointestinal disorders tend to be less aware of their possible significance in the treatment of serum cholesterol problems. As bad as many of our 'civilized' diets are, the use of a non-toxic nutrient agent as an aid in efforts to keep cholesterol levels within a reasonable range certainly seems a logical step.

While cholesterol is an important component found in every cell membrane in your body, and without it normal metabolic processes would be impossible, an excessive level of cholesterol in the blood (hypercholesterolaemia) is considered to be a major health risk. It is one of the main factors leading to the development of atherosclerosis.

The higher the levels of low density lipoprotein (LDL) cholesterol in the bloodstream the faster atherosclerosis develops. High density lipoprotein (HDL) is found in plentiful supplies in people with low incidence of atherosclerosis and, therefore, of good cardiac health. HDL plays an important part in actually removing excessive levels of cholesterol from tissues.

The liver actually manufactures far more cholesterol itself than is obtained through the diet. In fact, if the diet is rich in animal fats (meat and dairy products) the liver actually increases its own production of cholesterol.

The gall-bladder releases bile salts to help us digest the fats we eat. After being used in this manner the bile salts are broken down (by bifidobacteria), reabsorbed from the small intestine and are returned to the liver for re-use or are eliminated in the feces.

Excessive quantities of bile salts (as in a fat-rich diet) damage or inhibit the bifidobacteria (as well as numerous other bacterial inhabitants of the colon). This is one more good reason for avoiding a high fat diet.

Research by several different groups of scientists suggests that probiotic L. acidophilus has a possible role in lowering serum cholesterol and low density lipoproteins (LDL). (Mohan, Schauss)

The intestinal tract has a major effect on cholesterol metabolism. This is the site where cholesterol is absorbed. The bacterial population in the intestine greatly impacts the degree of absorption and cholesterol synthesis. Dietary supplements and probiotics have a variable effect on plasma cholesterol concentrations. (Salminen)

Research shows that there must be an anti-cholesterolemic milk factor (AMF) in the fermented milk which seems to inhibit an enzyme which synthesizes cholesterol in the liver. Similar anticholesterolemic effects have now been demonstrated from constituents of live yogurt.

Both animal and human studies now show that cultured milk products such as yogurt and acidophilus milk, efficiently lower levels of cholesterol in the blood. (Anderson, Brashears, Buck, Gilliland)

Researchers state that this reduction could be because of alteration in cholesterol synthesis, absorption, conversion into bile acids or the synthesis and breakdown of lipoprotein. No firm conclusions have been reached.

It is established however, that the selection of the organism in a probiotic supplement has a significant impact on its ability to affect cholesterol levels.

It is not our intent to suggest the use of probiotics as a cure for the world's cholesterol problems, but it's pretty exciting that this remarkable supplement is so versatile and important.

Probiotics and the Immune System

Potential immune system benefits of lactic acid bacteria include:

- Stimulate antibody production with a wide range of antimicrobial activity against common food-borne pathogens (Pelto)
- Increase phagocytic and lymphocytic activity (Pelto, Perdigon,1988)
- Regulate immunity - stimulate it in healthy individuals and down-regulation of immunoinflammatory response in milk-hypersensitive subjects (Pelto)
- Prevent chemically induced tumors (Reddy, Naidu, Gallaher, Rowland)
- Protect against enteric infections
- Modify cytokine production (Pelto)
- Increase immunity by reducing malnutrition

Probiotics can increase immunoglobulins in the body, which seek out and destroy undesirables. IgA is known to increase. Studies show yogurt may inhibit the growth of intestinal carcinoma through increased activity of IgA, T cells, and macrophages. (Perdigon)

Animals fed with fermented milk showed an increase in both phagocytic and lymphocytic activity after 3 days. Mice fed lactic acid cultures demonstrated increased levels of macrophages and polymorphonucleases (as indicators of nonspecific immune response) and B and T lymphocytes (as indicators of humoral immune response). (Perdigon, 1989)

A protective mechanism of the probiotics themselves is to produce their own antibiotics, as a defense for their own survival. We can benefit from these antibiotics as well.

Specific strains of acidophilus are known to produce a natural antibiotic, which has been shown to possess a wide range of antimicrobial activity against common food-borne pathogens. The following organisms can be inhibited by this natural antibiotic:

Bacillus subtilis
Bacillus cereus
Bacillus stearothermophilus
Streptococcus faecalis var. liquifaciens
Pseudomonas fluorescens
Pseudomonas aeruginosa
Serratia marcescens
Salmonella schottmuelleri
Escherichia coli
Lactobacillus plantarum
Lactobacillus leichmannii
Lactobacillus lactis
Lactobacillus casei
Salmonella typhosa
Shigella dysenteriae
Shigella paradysenteriae
Staphylococcus aureus
Streptococcus lactis
Sarcina lutea
Klebsiella pneumoniae
Proteus vulgaris
Vibrio comma

Cancer

It is commonly known that we are forming cancerous cells in our bodies all the time. Ideally the immune systems recognizes this event and acts accordingly, attacking and eliminating the abnormal cell. Therefore, anything that is known to enhance the immune system is indirectly protecting us against cancer.

The actual formation of tumors (benign and malignant) requires two phases - initiation and promotion. There must be some cause of the abnormal formation of the cells in the first place. This alone, however, is not enough to give you the actual disease. The required environment must be present to allow these cells to adequately reproduce such that they can take over the surrounding tissue area. Without that you avoid the signs and symptoms that we recognize as a cancer.

There are several reports of the ability of probiotics to not only help prevent cancer, but actually act to inhibit the growth of cancers. (Reddy, Naidu, Gallaher, Rowland)

Methods by which it does this include:

- Inhibits mutagenic activity;
- Decreases several enzymes which create carcinogens, mutagens, or tumor-promoting agents;
- Suppresses tumor growth;
- Supports the immune system (controls cell-mediated immune responses, activates reticuloendothelial system, augments cytokine pathways and regulates interleukins, and tumor necrosis factors. (Naidu)

By reducing levels of enzymes that convert procarcinogens to actual carcinogens the incidence of cancer can be greatly reduced. The colon serves as an excellent host for potentially carcinogenic agents - thus one of the reasons for the common problem of colon cancer.

Other researchers have discovered similar results, both in the supplement's ability to lower amounts of procarcinogens, and its ability to stimulate immune response against tumor activity. (Roe, Modler, Hughes)

In humans, colon, cervical and breast cancers have been specifically mentioned. Select strains of acidophilus and bifidus have specific activity against certain tumors. (Rao-colon, McNicol-cervix, Rice-breast)

Goldin and Gorbach have found indications that proper intestinal flora are worthwhile, both by helping other factors control the formation of carcinogens, and by actually lowering the incidence of chemically-induced tumors in animal studies. (Goldin)

Probiotics May Help Prevent Colon Cancer

Colorectal cancer is a major disease of Western civilizations and diet may account for at least 35% of cases. Epidemiologic studies reveal that the major dietary constituents implicated in the disease process are fat/red meat (causative) and fibre (protective).

Researchers in New York examined the potential anticancer properties of two different concentrations of L.

acidophilus in laboratory animals. Their results showed that the animals with probiotic supplementation significantly suppressed precancerous and suspicious cells. L. acidophilus inhibited cancerous cell formation in a dose-dependent manner.

These results suggest that L. acidophilus may potentially prevent colon cancer development. Further studies are warranted in humans to determine the full potential of this probiotic strain in preclinical efficacy studies. (Rao)

Researchers in the UK also found that probiotic consumption was also associated with decreases in factors that have been associated with carcinogenesis of the colon in experimental animal models. (Rowland)

Probiotics Help Protect Against Radiation Affects

The ability of probiotics to protect against the effects of radiation logically offer protection against the endpoint of radiation damage - and it's not limited just to the colon area. Select strains have the ability to help protect against the overall deleterious effects of therapeutic radiation (and chemotherapy) in conventional cancer treatments.

Probiotic bacteria are used to treat disturbed intestinal microflora and increased gut permeability which are characteristic to many intestinal disorders. Examples include children with acute rotavirus diarrhea, subjects with food allergy, subjects with colonic disorders and patients undergoing pelvic radiotherapy and sometimes changes associated with colon cancer development. In all such disease states, altered intestinal microflora, impaired gut barrier and different types of intestinal inflammation are present.

Proper probiotic bacteria are able to survive gastric conditions and colonize the intestine, at least temporarily, by adhering to the intestinal tract. Existing preparations containing viable lactic bacteria of human origin appear to have value in restoring normal microbial functions and alleviating symptoms in some patients with gastrointestinal infection and other conditions. (Strus)

Other Benefits of Probiotics

Arthritis

Rheumatoid arthritis has a link to the use of probiotics. Specific harmful bacterial overgrowths in the GI tract have been linked to arthritic diseases, including ankylosing spondylitis, and the ability to kill these bacteria with beneficial organisms has been established. Benefits of this type of treatment, along with a diet that is friendly to healthy flora have been shown in human clinical studies.

Finish researchers reported that large amounts of living lactobacilli consumed daily may also have positive effects on objective measures of rheumatoid arthritis. (Nenonen)

Animal studies show that certain mice prone to develop collagen (CII)-induced arthritis (CIA), who are orally given a certain strain of L. acidophilus (Shirota) in their drinking water experience a reduced incidence of CIA compared to controls. The treated mice also tested fewer CIA-specific antibodies and suppressed the CII-specific secretion of interferon-gamma. The treated mice who did develop CIA, also experienced a delayed response compared to controls. From these results, the researchers concluded that the Lactobacillus was able to modify the humoral and cellular immune responses to CII, and these modifications could result in the reduction of the development of CIA. (Kato)

Acne and other Skin Problems

Italian researchers have reported evidence that regulating intestinal bacterial flora may be an effective therapy of for acne vulgaris, an adult skin disorder. (Marchetti)

Jonathan V. Wright, M.D., perhaps the foremost

nutritional therapist in the world, has found a link between constipation, low stomach acidity, and acne rosacea, sometimes called "adult acne" to distinguish it from "teenage acne". It is characterized by an increase in size and visibility of the blood vessels under the skin of the nose, chin and forehead, causing a bright red appearance.

Dr. Wright feels that acidophilus and probiotics are even more important than another part of his therapy, adding digestive enzymes and hydrochloric acid. Benefits have also been seen in other skin problems, such as eczema and psoriasis.

Liver Health

Liver failure is a serious condition. The liver has hundreds of important functions and responsibilities-one of which is to keep ammonia levels in the blood down to an acceptable level. Rising levels of ammonia in the system can cause a disorder called hepatic (liver) encephalopathy, a serious brain disease. This can result in disturbed states of consciousness and behavior, tremors, and may even progress to full coma.

As far back as the 1960's it was known that observable clinical improvement was possible in patients with this disease, due to the ammonia-lowering effects of probiotics. Harvard researchers found that probiotics helped both mental confusion and overall clinical status.

Researchers at the Department of Pathology, New England Deaconess Hospital, Boston, MA, demonstrated in laboratory animals that L. acidophilus feeding reduces endotoxemia and severity of experimental alcoholic liver disease and reduces the degree of alcoholic liver damage. The researchers concluded that L. acidophilus provides a potential nontoxic form of therapy for both endotoxemia and alcoholic liver disease. (Nanji)

This has also been confirmed in a human study with 35 patients with alcohol cirrhosis. They were treated orally with Bifidobacterium bifidum and L. acidophilus for several months. Thirty cirrhotics were treated for the same length of time with lactulose and diuretics. Bifidobacterium bifidum/L. acidophilus-treated patients showed reduced ammonium levels, improvement of mental status and psychological performance. In addition, patients who required hospitalization had shorter in-patient periods thanks to a more rapid psychological and physical improvement. The researchers concluded that probiotics may be considered a valid alternative to conventional therapy for the out-patient management of subjects with alcoholic cirrhosis. (Colle)

Kidney Health

Japanese researchers demonstrated that lactic acid bacteria help inhibit accumulation of toxins in the blood of patients with kidney failure. These toxins, naturally produced in the intestine as bacterial putrefactive metabolites, are normally filtered out of the blood by the kidneys. Plasma levels of uremic toxins (phenol, p-cresol, and indican) are markedly increased in kidney failure patients, and cannot be efficiently reduced by dialysis. The results in the study demonstrated that oral administration of lactic acid bacteria in these patients is effective in reducing the levels of these toxins, especially that of indican, in the blood by inhibiting bacterial production by means of correcting the intestinal microflora. (Hida)

Probiotics are also helpful for:

Bacterial Vaginosis: Take probiotic supplements orally and through intravaginal douche.

Recurrent Bladder Infections: Take probiotic supplements orally.

Prebiotics

Probiotics, defined as microbial food supplements that beneficially affect the host by improving its intestinal microbial balance, have been used to change the composition of colonic microbiota. However, such changes may be transient, and the implantation of exogenous bacteria therefore becomes limited.

In contrast, **pre**biotics are nondigestible food ingredients that beneficially affect the host by selectively stimulating the growth and/or activity of one or a limited number of bacterial species already resident in the colon, and thus attempt to improve host health. Intake of prebiotics can significantly increase the number of specific bacteria and thus change the composition of the microbiota. Nondigestible oligosaccharides, fructooligosaccharides (FOS), and inulin (selective fermentable chicory fructan), are examples of prebiotics. Many of these are long chain sugar molecules. (Reddy, 1999)

Prebiotics stimulate the growth of endogenous bifidobacteria. Prebiotics also modulate lipid metabolism, most likely via fermentation products. By combining the rationale of pro- and prebiotics, the concept of ***symbiotics*** is proposed to characterize some colonic foods with interesting nutritional properties that make these compounds candidates for classification as health-enhancing functional food ingredients. (Gibson)

Prebiotics Benefit Metabolism

In animals, FOS suppresses production of triglycerides and VLDL in the liver, resulting in marked reductions in triglyceride and cholesterol levels. (Taylor, Roberfroid)

In adult diabetics, it lowers both cholesterol and fasting blood sugar levels by significant amounts, while similar amounts of common table sugar had no such effect.

In conclusion, FOS can help correct problems in both carbohydrate and fat metabolism in these individuals.

Prebiotics Help Prevent Colon Cancer

Laboratory studies show that dietary administration of prebiotics (oligofructose and inulin) inhibits the formation of precancerous lesions in the colon suggesting the potential colon tumor inhibitory properties. Higher levels of bifidobacteria and tumor inhibitory activities, result in inhibition of colon carcinogenesis, and a decrease in colonic mucosal cell proliferation and tumor activities. (Reddy)

Fructooligosaccharides (FOS)

FOS is a naturally-occurring prebiotic compound found in many edible sources such as artichokes, bananas, honey, onion, garlic, barley, and others. It is non-toxic, and has few side effects. (It can cause bowel gas when rapidly introduced into an uninitiated GI tract.) It has been used as a food item in Japan for years, and is a feed additive for poultry in the U.S. (Spiegel)

FOS represents a very special type of sugar. It does taste sweet, though not as sweet as common table sugar, but the difference is well worth it. The significance is that probiotic bacteria can readily utilize FOS to vastly and quickly increasing their numbers. (Yamazaki, Hartemink)

The ever-present invading bacteria and yeast in our environment do not have enzymes necessary to break down this potential energy source. If they can't metabolize it, they can't use it for food, while the probiotic bacteria can. If the diet is well-controlled in terms of sugar and other refined carbohydrates, acidophilus can aggressively multiply while invaders are having trouble just finding something to eat!

In addition, FOS have additional nutritional properties on digestive physiological parameters like colonic pH and stool bulking which justify their classification as dietary fibers. It has also been reported that they improve the bioavailability of essential minerals. (Roberfroid)

What's more, for the diet-conscious, is that humans cannot absorb and metabolize FOS either. This means we can obtain all it's advantages of rapid probiotic proliferation, while not increasing caloric intake.

Selection Criteria For Probiotic Supplements

All probiotic products are not alike and do not have similar nutritional and therapeutic values. The name probiotic does not mean anything unless it contains the right strain, in the right amount, in the right formulation and in the right condition (viable) for the intended use.

For this reason one needs to know the strain, its viability, implantation criteria, its other features and health benefits.

All probiotic supplements are not alike and do not have similar nutritional and therapeutic values. The name probiotic does not mean anything unless it contains the right strain, in the right amount, in the right formulation and in the right condition (viable) for the intended use.

For this reason one has to know the strain, its viability, implantation criteria, its other features and health benefits.

Strain Selection

Lactic acid bacteria have long history of their safe use in dairy products. However, some novel probiotic supplements now contain bacteria which have no safe use record in human or animal food supplements or foods. There are instances of probiotic supplements containing soil bacteria which are not normal inhabitants of human gastrointestinal tract and can be of pathogenic potential. It is imperative to select the bacteria for incorporation in probiotic supplements which are in the GRAS (Generally Recognized As Safe) list. For example, Lactobacillus acidophilus species and some Bifidobacterium species are considered GRAS.

Any new bacterial culture which has no history of prior safe use in humans, should be subject to toxicological studies prior to incorporation in any probiotic supplements.

The bacterial strains used in the probiotic supplements should play an important role in:

- Colonization resistance in the intestinal, respiratory and urogenital tracts
- Cholesterol metabolism
- Inhibiting the carcinogenesis, directly or indirectly, by stimulation of immune system
- The metabolism of lactose, the absorption of calcium and the synthesis of vitamins
- Reduction of yeast and vaginal infection
- Constipation and diarrheal diseases
- Gastritis and ulcers
- Acne and skin problems
- Adherence and colonization of microorganisms used in probiotic supplement is a very important criteria in the selection of probiotic supplements.
- Probiotic strain to survive stomach acid
- The production of natural antibiotics, lactic acid and hydrogen peroxide and inhibiting the pathogenic bacteria such as:

Bacillus xubtilis
Bacillus cereus
Bacillus stearothermophilus
Streptococcus faecalis
Streptococcus faecalis var liquifaciens
Streptococcus lactis
Lactobacillus lactis
Lactobacillus casei
Lactobacillus plantarum
Lactobacillus leichmannii
Sarcina lutea
Serratia marcescens
Proteus vulgaris
Escherichia coli
Salmonella typhosa
Salmonella schottmuelleri
Shigella dysenteriae
Shigella paradysenteriae
Psuedomonas fluorescens
Pseudomonas aeruginosa
Staphylococcus aureus
Lkebsiella pneumoniae
Vibrio comma

Source: US Patent #3,689,640 In Vitro Antibacterial Activity of DDS-1 Lactobacillus Acidophilus

Not all strains of Lactobacillus acidophilus and other probiotics are acid-resistant. Selecting acid-resistant strains of L acidophilus and other probiotics is the key to the success of the probiotic supplement. This assures the survival of the probiotics in the stomach acid which are usually acidic.

Probiotic supplements with multiple bacteria

Some novel probiotic supplements now contain many bacteria which have no safe use history in human health and nutrition. These bacteria may be antagonistic to each other and may alter the gut flora in an undesirable way.

So it should not be believed that if one bacterium is good, two are better and many are best!

L. acidophilus and Bifidobacterium species are normal inhabitants of human gastrointestinal tract and are GRAS. Probiotic formulations containing these beneficial bacteria along with prebiotic fructooligosaccharides (FOS) are considered safe and offer many health benefits described earlier.

Manufacturing

The manufacturing process used to produce microorganisms for use in probiotic supplements plays an important role. The medium, the temperature and other associated factors influence the viability and identity of the microorganisms. If the probiotic supplements do not contain the same microorganisms with the same viability, they will not offer the same consistent good results.

Also make sure that the probiotic culture has not been contaminated with other harmful bacteria during manufacturing process and packaging.

Viability

- The decrease of viability of probiotics is also strain-dependent and also influenced strongly by their physiochemical environment.

- Probiotics in liquid medium including milk, yogurt do not normally survive longer than three days to two weeks.

- Exposure of probiotics to oxygen decrease the stability of probiotic bacteria.

● Eliminating oxygen from and including nitrogen into probiotic supplement bottles can enhance the stability of probiotics.

Guarantee/Assay

It is also very important that the probiotic supplements are tested for the type and number of viable microorganisms at the manufacturing and at the expiration date. This quality control procedure is important to the manufacturer as well as the consumer.

The viable cells are guaranteed as CFU (colony forming units) per gram at the time of probiotic supplement packaging. Consumption of probiotic supplements with two to five billion CFU per day is necessary to have any chance of offering any beneficial effects.

Storage, Handling and Shipping

Storage of probiotic supplements at 40oF is recommended to maintain the viability of the microorganisms and used prior to the expiration date of the product (All probiotic supplements must bear expiration date). Probiotic supplements, if not kept refrigerated, may not have viable microorgnisms.

Probiotic supplements should be shipped in insulated containers via air freight to avoid exposure to heat. Viability will not decline with short exposure to heat during shipping. Some companies package probiotic supplements in nitrogen-flushed bottles to maintain viability of the microorganisms during shipping and handling. Also the supplements contain higher potency (higher CFU) than guaranteed on the label.

Glass Bottle vs. Plastic Bottle

Probiotics are "anaerobic" organisms, meaning they live in the absence of oxygen. Therefore, exposure to air is undesirable. This makes glass a preferred container over plastic, which is somewhat porous. Probiotics packaged in plastic bottles can lose its potency to some degree.

Dairy vs. Non-Dairy

Some candida specialists recommend that individuals who are allergic to dairy products should consume non-dairy probiotic supplements for better results.

Prebiotic/Probiotic Combinations

Combination of prebiotics with probiotics offer better opportunities to the probiotic strains to grow and multiply faster in the gastrointestinal tract as prebiotics selectively feed probiotics.

Capsule, Tablets, Powder or Liquid?

Capsules are preferred over powder. Some individuals find it difficult to measure exact dosages with the powder. In addition, each time the powder bottle is opened, the contents are exposed to atmospheric contamination. The powder is oxidized, and is exposed to humidity as well as to the contaminants. The spoon used to measure the powder may also add to the contamination if it is not sterile, as well as adding moisture to the powder. For these reasons, deterioration of powder tends to be more rapid when compared to capsules and tablets.

- Capsules add another layer of insulation against these conditions. Capsules are most preferred by consumers.

- Chewable Tablets are acceptable (and often preferred by children). It is vegetarian. Older people prefer to use tablets as some cannot swallow and they keep it under the tongue, and it dissolves.

- Liquid Probiotics do not normally survive longer than three days to two weeks. Another disadvantage is that microorganisms in liquid medium can mutate and change.

How and When to Use Probiotic Supplements

Excessive use of antibiotics, chlorinated water, processed and junk foods, and polluted environment reduce the number of friendly bacteria in the gastrointestinal tract. Seventy percent of women and forty percent of men have yeast infection and lack probiotics in their gut. The studies at the VA Hospital of Minneapolis show normal persons have almost no probiotics in their gastrointestinal tracts. For this reason, it is advisable that one should take a proven probiotic supplement daily.

Probiotic supplements containing L. acidophilus, Bifidobacterium species and FOS with two to five billion live cells (2 – 5 x 109 CFU) should be taken daily just before breakfast or between meals for maintenance.

Health professionals recommend probiotic supplements for candidiasis (yeast infection), digestive disorders (including diarrhea and constipation), gastritis, lactose intolerance, gas, heartburn, irritable bowel, colitis, crohn's disease and immune disfunctions and as a follow up to antibiotic therapy. Under these conditions higher amounts of the probiotic supplements are used.

Remember, if the probiotic supplements are not refrigerated and viable, they will offer no health benefits. Also, if these supplements are not taken in sufficient quantities, they will produce no results.

Reminder: Use of probiotic supplements or any other supplements should be taken with the advice of a health professional who has knowledge and expertise in probiotics and other supplements.

DDS® Acidophilus

DDS® Acidophilus is the brand manufactured by UAS Laboratories, 5620 Rowland Rd., Minnetonka, MN 55343 (800-422-3371), who has been researching probiotic supplements even before its inception in 1979. DDS® is a rice-based supplement, producing a strain researched to have superior attributes. (Sehnert)

An additional attribute includes it's ability to survive stomach acid, allowing colonization farther along the GI tract. (Sehnert) UAS products do need such protection so can be used as powder, gelatin capsules, or chewable. Studies at the VA Hospital in Minneapolis confirm this. (Sehnert)

Research done by Lance R. Peterson, M.D., Chief, Infectious Diseases Section of the Veteran's Administration Medical Center, Minneapolis, MN, showed stability of DDS® Acidophilus in the digestive system. He stated, "*The general impression I have from this study is that those patients upon whom we received pre-and during-therapy specimens increased their numbers of lactobacilli more than one-hundredfold in their stool. I would conclude that this gives evidence that the organisms were able to persist and likely replicate during the transition of the gut in these studied patients.*"

For maximal effect, the best production of bacteria killing chemicals is supremely important in strain selection. DDS is known to have high amounts of lactic acid, hydrogen peroxide, and natural antibiotics, in a powerful selection.

The correct mixture of different types of bacteria, like L. acidophilus and bifidus is very important as competition between different organisms can lower the strength from what was originally put in the bottle. UAS has closely studied these effects to avoid such problems.

In addition, UAS mixes the bacteria in a base of FOS to encourage proliferation where needed in the body.

During a three-month interval, Dr. Keith Sehnert provided DDS® Acidophilus to 42 patients at a primary care clinic. Here are some of the responses reported in response cards they returned. Some had more than one improvement.

Reduced candida symptoms 22
Corrected digestive disorders 21
Decreased constipation 15
Decreased bad breath 7
Improved acne problems 6
Other improvements 5

The Surprising Story Behind Probiotics

During the past few years, people have been increasingly using probiotics to supplement their diets and bolster their immune system while on antibiotics. Also, probiotics are used for yeast infection, diarrhea, acne, high cholesterol and other ailments. How did probiotics find their way from a dusty, hidden shelf to mainstream modern medicine?

From 1973 to 1979, Dr. S.K. Dash was Director of the Food and Drug Program for the state of South Dakota. While reviewing and licensing veterinary products, he discovered that a probiotic product was approved as a drug in the 1970s and sold by a major pharmaceutical company. Dr. Dash also uncovered the fact that probiotics have been 97% effective in combating E. coli infection in pigs, as was the antibiotic Neomycin Sulfate.

So what happened to the great probiotic products? Dr. Dash found that big pharmaceutical companies used millions of dollars in research, development, marketing and promotion and took over the market with antibiotics—the miracle drug of the time. Probiotic firms lacked funds to compete with drug firms in research, development, marketing and promotions and lost the battle against antibiotic manufacturers.

Over the past 15 years, the health trend has shifted from prescription to nutrition. More people are looking for nutritional and natural supplements as an answer to their problems. People are concerned about the quality of their environment, water, food and the side effects of the medication they take.

Dr. Dash was among the first to answer these concerns in 1979 when he founded UAS Labs. Dr. Dash said that with his extensive knowledge in probiotics, "I decided to leave my secure state government job and start an innovative and technology driven company to lead the probiotic concept." According to Dr. Dash, the market reacted positively to his company and product right from the start.

"*DDS® Acidophilus was well accepted,*" he said. "*UAS Laboratories developed the first non-dairy acidophilus – a refrigerated item – and packaged it in nitrogen-flushed glass bottles. This helped UAS set quality standards for probiotic products. An ongoing quality assurance program helps to maintain the high quality of his company's products*, Dr. Dash said. "*We have an unrelenting commitment to quality,*" he said. "*When we put out any product, we guarantee it will be the best available quality.*"

Dr. Dash was the first to set a quality control standard for probiotics by requiring guarantees of CFU (Colony Forming Units) on probiotic product labels. The lists of other "first" for UAS Labs, according to Dr. Dash, include being the first company to offer non-dairy acidophilus, the first to introduce chewable vegan tablets, the first to introduce nitrogen packaging, and the first to incorporate FOS in probiotic products.

UAS Laboratories is the first in commercially manufacturing and marketing the super-strain, DDS-Acidophilus and DDS-Plus.

The philosophy of UAS Labs, Dr. Dash noted, is "*to be an innovative and technology driven company dedicated to promoting healthy living by providing superior quality probiotic products and other nutritional supplements.*"

Bibliography

Aiba Y, et al. Lactic acid-mediated suppression of Helicobacter pylori by the oral administration of Lactobacillus salivarius as a probiotic in a gnotobiotic murine model. Am J Gastroenterol. 1998 Nov;93(11):2097-101.

Alm L; Acidophilus milk for therapy in gastrointestinal disorders. Nahrung 1984;28(6-7):683-4

Alm, L.; The effect of Lactobacillus acidophilus administration upon the survival of Salmonella in randomly selectly human carriers. Prog. Food Nutr. Sci., 1983, 7:13-17.

Alm L, Effect of fermentation on lactose, glucose, and galactose content in milk and suitability of fermented milk products for lactose intolerant individuals. J Dairy Sci. 1982 Mar;65(3):346-52.

Alm L, The effect of fermentation on the biological value of milk proteins evaluated using rats. A study on Swedish fermented milk products. J Sci Food Agric. 1981 Dec;32(12):1247-53.

Anderson JW; Gilliland SE; Effect of fermented milk (yogurt) containing Lactobacillus acidophilus L1 on serum cholesterol in hypercholesterolemic humans. J Am Coll Nutr 1999 Feb;18(1):43-50.

Atkinson-Barr, M., Marshall. B.; "Halitosis and H. pylori: A Case Study", Helicobacter Web.,1996, p.1.

Bagchi, Dash, *Natural Antibiotics and Beyond*, Townsend Letter For Doctor's and Patients,Feb/Mar. 1996.

Brashears MM; Gilliland SE; Buck LM; Bile salt deconjugation and cholesterol removal from media by Lactobacillus casei. J Dairy Sci 1998 Aug;81(8):2103-10.

Buck, L, et al; Comparisons of Freshly isolated strains of L acidophilus of human intestinal origin for ability to assimilate cholesterol during growth. J Dairy Science, 1994; 77:2925-2933.

Campieri M; Gionchetti P; Probiotics in inflammatory bowel disease: new insight to pathogenesis or apossible therapeutic alternative? [editorial; comments] Gastroenterology 1999 May;116(5):1246-9

Clements,M.L, et al; Exogenour lactobacili fed to men: Their fate and ability to prevent diarrheal disease. Prog Food Nutr. 1983, 7, 29-37.

Colle R; Ceschia T; Oral bacteriotherapy with Bifidobacterium bifidum and Lactobacillus acidophilus in cirrhotic patients] Clin Ter 1989 Dec 31;131(6):397-402.

Collins MD; Gibson GR; Probiotics, prebiotics, and synbiotics: approaches for modulating the microbial ecology of the gut. Am J Clin Nutr 1999 May;69(5):1052S-1057S.

Crook,W; The Yeast Connection, Prof. Books., 1986.

Elmer et al; Biotherapeutic Agents, A Neglected Modality, JAMA,1996: 275:870-876.

Favier C; Neut C; Mizon C; Cortot A; Colombel JF; Mizon J; Fecal beta-D-galactosidase production and Bifidobacteria are decreased in Crohn's disease. Dig Dis Sci 1997 Apr;42(4):817-22.

Fiedorek, S.C. et al, Fastors influencing the epidemiology of H. pylori infection in children. Ped, 1991,88 578-82.

Fitzsimmons,et al.; Inhibition of Candida albicans by L. acidophilus, Microbios,1994, Vol 80;125-133.

Gallaher DD; Khil J; The effect of synbiotics on colon carcinogenesis in rats. Department of Food Science and Nutrition, University of Minnesota, St. Paul, MN J Nutr 1999 Jul;129(7 Suppl):1483S-7S.

Gibson GR; Roberfroid MB; Dietary modulation of the human colonic microbiota: introducing the concept of prebiotics.. J Nutr 1995 Jun;125(6):1401-12.

Gilliland, S, et al; Assimilation of cholesterol by lactobabillus acidophilus. Applied and Environmental Microbiology, 1985;49:2, 377-381.

Goldin BR; Health benefits of probiotics. Department of Family Medicine and Community Health, TuftsUniversity School of Medicine, Boston, MA, Br J Nutr 1998 Oct;80(4):S203-7

Golz. V. et al; Prolylaxis againstampicillian-associated diarrhea with a lactobacillus preparation. Amer. J. Hosp. Pharmacol., 1979, 36, 754.

Gorbach, S.L. Goldin, B.R.; Nutrition and the Gastrointestinal Microflora, Nutrition Review, 1992, Vol. 50: 12, 378-381.

Haenel, H., Benedig, J.; Intestinal flora in health and diseasem Amer. J Clin Nutr.,1970, 1, 21-64.

Hartemink R; Rombouts FM; Comparison of media for the detection of bifidobacteria, lactobacilli and total anaerobes from faecal samples. J Microbiol Methods 1999 Jun;36(3):181-92.

Hida M; Aiba Y; Sawamura S; Suzuki N; Satoh T; Koga Y; Inhibition of the accumulation of uremic toxins in the blood and their precursors in the feces after oral administration of Lebenin, a lactic acid bacteria preparation, to uremic patients undergoing hemodialysis. Nephron 1996;74(2):349-55.

Hilton, et al, Ingestion of Yogurt as Prophylaxis for Oandidal Vaginitis', Ann. Int Med.,1992:116; 353-357.

Hitchins, A.D., et al;Amelioration of the adverse effect of a gastrointestinal challenge woth Salmonellaenteritidis on weanling rats by a yogurt culture diet. Amer. J Clin Nutr. 1985, 41, 41-100.

Hove H; Norgaard H; Mortensen PB Lactic acid bacteria and the human gastrointestinal tract Eur J Clin Nutr 1999 May;53(5):339-50.

Hughes. D., Hoover D; Bifidobacteria, Food Technology, April 1991, 76-78.

Lykova EA; Bondarenko VM; et al; Combined antibacterial and probiotic therapy of Helicobacter- associated diseases inchildren. Zh Mikrobiol Epidemiol Immunobiol 1999 Mar-Apr;(2):76-8.

Kato, I, et al; Suppressive effects of the oral administration of Lactobacillus casei on type II collagen-induced arthritis in DBA/1 mice. Life Sci. 1998; 63(8):635-44.

Kim, H.S; Gilliland, S.E.; Lactobacillus acidophilus as a dietary adjunct for milk to aid lactose digestion in humans, J Dairy Sci, 1983; 66, 959-66.

Kolars, J.C. et al; Yogurt- an autodigesting source of lactose. New Engl. J. Med. 1984, 310, 1-3

Kruis, W; Schutz E; Fric P; Fixa B; et al. Double-blind comparison of an oral Escherichia coli preparation and mesalazine in maintaining remission of ulcerative colitis. Aliment Pharmacol Ther 1997 Oct;11(5): 853-8

Madsen, KL; Doyle, JS et al; Lactobacillus species prevents colitis in interkeukin 10 gene-deficient mice, Gastroenterology, 1999, May;116(5);1246-9.

Majamaa, H. A novel approach in the management of food allergy, J Aller Olin Immunol, 1997 Feb;99(2):179-85.

Marchetti, F, et al. Efficacy of regulators of the intestinal bacterial flora in the therapy of acne vulgaris. Clin Ter. 1987 Sep 15;122(5):339-43.

McDonough, F.E. et al; Modification of sweet acidolphulus milk to improve ultilization by lactose-intolerant persons. Amer J Clin Nutr, 1987, 45, 570-4.

McGrory, et al, 'Interaction of L. acidopholis and T. vaginalis in vitro, J. Parisitol., 80 (1), 1994, 50-54.

McNicol, PJ; Paraskevas M; Guijon FB; The effect of vaginal microbes on in vivo and in vitro expression of human papillomavirus 16 E6-E7 genes. Cancer Detect Prev 1999;23(1):13-21.

Metchnikoff, E, The Prolongation of Life. Arna Press, NY. 1908 (1977 reprint)

Midolo, et al, J App Bac , 1995; 79, 478.

Mitsuoka Bifidobacteria and Their Role in Human Health, J. Indus. Micro. 1990, 6: 265.

Modler, H.W., et al.; Bifidobacteria and Bifidogenic Factors, Can. Inst. Food Sci., V.23, 1; 34.

Molin, G., Anderson, R. Ahrne, S., Lonner, C et al, Effect of fermented oatmeal soup on the cholesterol level and the Lactobacillus colonization of rat intestinal mucosa. Antonie can Leeuweenhoek, 1992; 61, 167-173.

Murray, F; Acidohilus and Your Health, Keats, 1998, 23-24.

Naidu, AS; Bidlack WR; Clemens RA; Probiotic spectra of lactic acid bacteria (LAB). College of Agriculture, California State Polytechnic University, Pomona. Crit Rev Food Sci Nutr 1999 Jan; 39(1):13-126.

Nanji, AA; Khettry, U; Sadrzadeh, SM; Lactobacillus feeding reduces endotoxemia and severity of experimental alcoholic liver (disease). Proc Soc Exp Biol Med 1994 Mar;205(3):243-7.

Nenonen, MT; Helve, TA; Rauma, AL; Uncooked, lactobacilli-rich, vegan food and rheumatoid arthritis. Br J Rheumatol 1998 Mar;37(3):274-81.

NIH Consensus Conference. H. pylori in Peptic Ulcer Disease, JAMA, 1994, Vol. 272:1, 65-69.

Noda. H.. et al.; Biotin Production by Bifidobacteria, J. Nutr. Sci. Vitaminol. 40, 181-188, 1994.

O'Sullivan, M.G. et al; Probiotic bacteria, myth or reality? Trends in Food Science and

Technology, 1992, 3: 309-14.

Pelto L; Isolauri E; Lilius EM; Nuutila J; Salminen S; Probiotic bacteria down-regulate the milk-induced inflammatory response in milk-hypersensitive subjects but have an immunostimulatory effect in healthy subjects. Turku, Finland. Clin Exp Allergy 1998 Dec;28(12):1474-9

Perdigon G; Alvarez S; Rachid M; Aguero G; Gobbato N; Immune system stimulation by probiotics. J Dairy Sci 1995 Jul;78(7):1597-606.

Perdigon G; de Macias ME; et al; Systemic augmentation of the immune response in mice by feeding fermented milks with Lactobacillus casei and Lactobacillus acidophilus. Immunology 1988 Jan;63(1):17-23.

Rao CV; Sanders ME; Indranie C; Simi B; Reddy BS; Prevention of colonic preneoplastic lesions by the probiotic Lactobacillus acidophilus NCFMTM in F344 rats. Int J Oncol 1999 May;14(5): 939-44.

Reddy BS; Prevention of colon cancer by pre- and probiotics: evidence from laboratory studies. American Health Foundation, Valhalla, New York 10595,J Nutr 1998 Oct;80(4):S219-23.

Reddy BS; Possible mechanisms by which pro- and prebiotics influence colon carcinogenesis and tumor growth. American Health Foundation, Valhalla, NY, J Nutr 1999 Jul;129(7 Suppl):1478S-82S.

Rice LJ, et al.; The effect of dietary fermented milk products and lactic acid bacteria on the initiation and promotion stages of mammary carcinogenesis. Nutr Cancer. 1995;24(2):99-109.

Roberfroid MB; Prebiotics and synbiotics: concepts and nutritional properties. Br J Nutr 1998 Oct;80(4):S197-202.

Roberfroid MB; Health benefits of non-digestible oligosaccharides. Department of Pharmaceutical Sciences, Universite Catholique de Louvain, Brussels, Belgium. Adv Exp Med Biol 1997;427:211-9.

Rotimi, V.O.; Duerden, B.I.; The development of the bacterial flora in normal neonates. J Med Microciol, 1974, 34, 51-62.

Rowland IR; Rumney CJ; et al; Effect of Bifidobacterium longum and inulin on gut bacterial metabolism and carcinogen-induced aberrant crypt foci in rats. Carcinogenesis 1998 Feb;19(2):281-5.

Salminen E., Elomaa, I. et al, PReservation of intestinal integrity during radiotherapy using live lactobacillus acidollhilus cultures. Clinical Radiotherapy, 1990, 39, 435-437.

Salminen S; Salminen E, Lactulose, lactic acid bacteria, intestinal microecology and mucosal protection.Dept. of Biochemistry and Food Chemistry, Turku University Hospital, Finland. Scand J Gastroenterol Suppl 1997;222:45-8

Saltzman JR, et al.; A randomized trial of Lactobacillus acidophilus BG2FO4 to treat lactose intolerance. Am J Clin Nutr. 1999 Jan;69(1):140-6.

Savaiano, D.A, et al; Lactose malabsorption from yogurt, pasteurized yogurt, sweet acidophulus milk and cultured milk in lactose-deficient individuals, Amer J Clin Nutr. 1984, 40, 12199-23.

Schauss, A.G. Lactobacillus acidophilus: Method of action, clinical application and toxicity data. Journ of Advan Med. 1990, 3; 163-178.

Siavoshi, F et al, Yeast: A Silent Companioan of H pylori which protects it against the environmental stresses. Gastro, 110: A1015, 1996.

Sehnert, K. The Gardin Within, Health World Magazine, Burlingame, CA. 1989.

Sghir A; Chow JM; Mackie RI; Continuous culture selection of bifidobacteria and lactobacilli from human faecal samples using fructooligosaccharide as selective substrate. J Appl Microbiol 1998 Oct;85(4):769-77.

Spiegel, et al.; Safety and Benefits of FOS as Food Ingredients, Food Technology, 1/94, p. 85.)

Stark, P.L., Lee, A.; The microbial ecology of the large bowel of breast-fed and formula-fed infants during the first year of life. J. Med. Microbial. 1982, 15, 189-203.

Strus M; The significance of lactic acid bacteria in treatment and prophylaxis of digestive tract disorders. Postepy Hig Med Dosw 1997;51(6):605-19.

Taylor GR; Williams CM; Effects of probiotics and prebiotics on blood lipids. Br J Nutr 1998 Oct;80(4):S225-30.

von Ritter C; Chronic inflammatory bowel diseases. Pathophysiology and drug therapy,1998 Jan;38(1):3-7.

Yamazaki, H, et al.; Meas. of Growth of Bifidobacteria, Let. in App. Micro., 1990,10, 229-232.

Index

About the Authors...

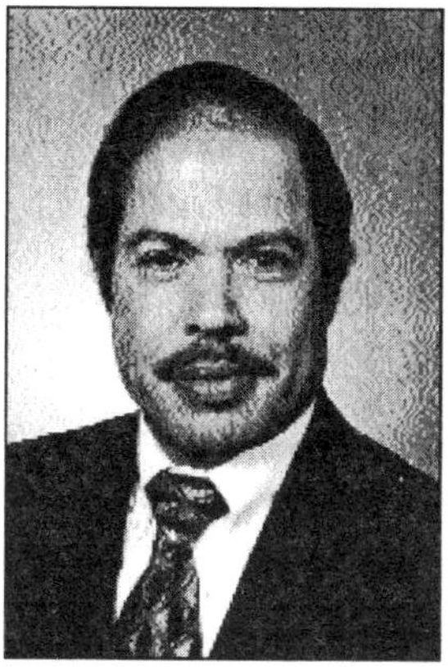

Dr. S.K. Dash received his Masters and Ph.D. degrees in Nutrition and Biochemistry from S.D. State University in 1970 and 1973. In that time he researched and published over 25 scientific papers in national and international journals. He immigrated to the US in 1969 from India.

From 1974-1980, Dr. Dash was a commissioned U.S. Food and Drug Administration Officer and Chairman of the Probiotic Products Committee (1975-1980). Dr. Dash has received several awards and honors for his pioneering work in probiotics.

Dr. Dash is currently the president and founder of UAS Laboratories, now located in Minnetonka, MN (1979). UAS is a biotech company specializing in probiotics and antioxidants. He is the developer of DDS® acidophilus and probiotic supplements holding the trademarks and proprietary formulas.

Dr. Allan N. Spreen is a licensed medical doctor who provides nutritional consulting and guidance to those seeking alternatives to conventional drug therapies. For over a decade he maintained a successful clinical nutrition practice in Jacksonville, Fl., where he was often featured on the local and radio talk shows. He has also served as an Olympic and U.S. National Diving Team Coach. Dr. Spreen is currently located in Arizona where he continues to write, lecture and consult full time to disseminate nutritional therapy information.

Dr. Beth M. Ley has been a science writer specializing in health and nutrition for over 12 years. She is the author/publisher of the Health Lerning Handbook series which currently lists over 10 titles. She received her B.S. degree in Scientific and Technical Writing from North Dakota State University in 1987 (combination of Zoology and Journalism). She also has her masters (1997) and doctoral degrees (1999) in Nutrition. Memberships include: American Academy of Anti-aging, New York Academy of Sciences and Oxygen Society.

YOU NEED TO KNOW...
THE HEALTH MESSAGE